HOW TO
SLIM
YOUR WAIST
FLATTEN
YOUR STOMACH &
TRIM
YOUR THIGHS
IN 30 DAYS

ABOUT THE AUTHOR

A southern Californian in heart and body, Katy Parks grew up in an environment in which health and fitness are a life style. She was a competitive athlete for 15 years and ran in several 10 kilometre and quarter-marathon races. She continues to run from 2–4 miles every day. She also swam competitively for 11 years.

Katy Parks' teaching career began as a swimming instructor at the YMCA and American Red Cross Association where she taught all levels of water skills, including life-saving, to all ages and also held classes for mentally and physically handicapped pupils. Her experience with disabilities came from over 6 years of working with deaf children at the California School for the Deaf.

Her interest in aerobic exercise began four years ago when she was introduced to the 'Jazzercise' method of dance-type workout. She now teaches at London's world-famous Pineapple Dance Studios where she holds her popular 'California Workout' routine consisting of aerobic and isometric exercises put to music.

ACKNOWLEDGEMENT

The cover photograph of Katy Parks and the photographs throughout the book are by Dick Makin; the line illustration is by Joanna Morrison.

All clothes worn by Katy Parks have been provided by Pineapple Dance Studios, 7 Langley Street, London W2. A mail order catalogue is available upon written request.

HOW TO SLIM YOUR WAIST FLATTEN YOUR STOMACH & TRIM YOUR THIGHS IN 30 DAYS

BY KATY PARKS

Arlington Books
Clifford Street Mayfair
London

HOW TO SLIM YOUR WAIST, FLATTEN YOUR STOMACH
AND TRIM YOUR THIGHS IN 30 DAYS
First published 1983 by
Arlington Books (Publishers) Ltd
3 Clifford Street Mayfair
London W1

Reprinted December 1983

© *Katy Parks 1983*

Typeset by Inforum Ltd, Portsmouth
Printed and bound by
The Richard Clay Group Ltd, Bungay

British Library Cataloguing in Publication Data
Parks, Katy
How to slim your waist, flatten your stomach and
trim your thighs in 30 days.
1. Exercise for women   2. Reducing exercises
I. Title
613.7'1   RA781.6

ISBN 0 85140 612 2

This book is dedicated to my flatmate,
Marina Sanchez-Elia, without whose advice,
understanding and TAB this book would never
have been written.

AN AVON SELF–CARE BOOK
FOR WOMEN
FROM ARLINGTON BOOKS

CONTENTS

INTRODUCTION

This book will show you how to slim your waist, flatten your stomach and trim your thighs in thirty days. It outlines a unique three-part programme – consisting of exercises, aerobics and advice on diet – that is guaranteed to work for you. By following the set routine you will discover a new power within – the kind of power that comes about only with control over your body.

The thirty-day programme contains a series of twelve exercises together with an aerobic sequence, both of which are explained simply and illustrated with photographs. The exercises have been specifically chosen to build up muscle flexibility and stamina, enhance freedom of movement, and strengthen the heart and lungs. You will burn off excess calories and reinvigorate the body – both physically and mentally.

Graduated charts at the back of the book will serve as a day-to-day itinerary with suggested repetitions. A drawing of the body, detailing all the muscles, is also included on page 13 which shows how the exercises will help to firm and tone the different parts of your body.

Both stretching and strengthening exercises have been incorporated into the routine, since it is most important that a balance be struck between the two disciplines. Extra-strong muscles that are never stretched become solid and short and thus ineffective. Conversely, stretching muscles without strengthening them causes loose ligaments and damaged joints, and muscles surrounding a joint must be strong to hold everything in place.

Special attention has also been given to warm-up and warm-down exercises. Warm-ups stretch and warm the muscles; they speed up blood circulation, promote relaxation and prepare the body for the more strenuous exercises of the routine. Warm-downs maintain the level of blood circulation so that the body is brought back to a resting temperature and allowed to cool gradually.

The warm-up and warm-down exercises reduce the risk of injury and soreness. They also enhance awareness of your muscles and, therefore, your body needs and capabilities. These exercises are essential parts of the programme and should never be eliminated.

Advice on diet follows the exercise and aerobic sections. Sensible eating is of paramount importance in order to achieve maximum fitness. Just as you cannot slim by diet alone, you cannot expect to lose weight by exercise alone. A calorie-controlled diet is essential.

A combined programme of regular exercise and sensible eating is really the *only* system of trimming that works. All muscular action has a physical consequence somewhere else, therefore you must strive for an harmonious balance of disciplines. Many people have followed the principles of my three-part programme with amazing results. You, too, will notice not only a difference in your waistline, but also in your face, your smile, your eyes.

Yes – exercising makes you vital. My three-part plan can make you vital too.

You have decided to tone your body. For whatever reason, you have decided that it is time to work on shaping those flabby thighs, flattening that bulging stomach and slimming that thickening waist. Fine. You have come to the right place. But, before you can begin you *must* understand what will be happening to your body in the process of toning. A brief explanation of your body's systematic and structural functions follows.

The body is an organic machine made up of living cells, all of which must be able to receive life-sustaining materials such as food and oxygen, and eliminate waste products such as carbon dioxide, urea and lactic acids. A system of transport, the circulatory system, has evolved which ensures that all the cells are reached. Blood, propelled by a muscular heart pump, flows through a closed tubular system of arteries, capillaries and veins, shunting the necessary materials.

One of the most important circuits in this system is the cardio-pulmonary. It circulates blood through the respiratory tissue of the lungs, picking up oxygen – the most vital, life-sustaining substance of the body. You can live without food or water for several days, but for only a few minutes without oxygen. At the same time, the cardio-pulmonary system removes waste products by releasing carbon dioxide and other gasses outside your body from your lungs. This process makes up the respiratory system and takes place both internally and externally.

External respiration is the exchange of gasses – oxygen and carbon dioxide – between the blood in your lungs' capillaries and alveoli. The alveoli are billions of tiny air chambers which are surrounded by the capillaries, minute branches of the blood vessels. The thin walls of these organelles allow for the gas exchange. Internal respiration is the exchange of the same gasses between your blood and tissues of your body cells.

Blood supply to every region and organ alters according to the oxygen needs of the moment. It is regulated by the contraction of your heart, heart beat and dilation of your arteries. For example, during muscular exercise, the arteries distributing to skeletal muscles dilate. At the same time, arteries supplying regions not in use are constricted. These responses are chemical reactions motivated by the metabolism of cells, that is, the transformation of food into energy. Thus, the more energy produced – speeding up your metabolism and production of chemicals – the more blood flows to your muscles and the faster you run. Your heart, unless it is flabby and out of shape, does not have to beat harder to keep up with the demand for more blood. The entire machine – you – runs more efficiently warmed in this way, and stays running efficiently hours after exercise.

As you can see, it is important that your heart and lungs always be in top working order to facilitate the rest of your body with its life supports. What is the point, for example, of a good set of tyres if the engine is weak? Aerobic exercises are especially helpful to enhance and strengthen your cardio-pulmonary capabilities and thus produce beneficial changes in your body. Any exercise that makes you work hard, demanding extra oxygen, is aerobic, or 'aerobian'.

Aerobic exercise strengthens and tones the heart itself and the 'intercostal muscles' which lie between the ribs and aid inhalation. It lowers blood pressure and heart rate by dilating the arteries, as well as stepping up your metabolism. Toning muscles improves circulation because

10

lean tissue is easier to pump through than fat. Your serum cholesterol also goes down. All these results aid in the prevention of coronary ailments. The debility of diabetes can be eased, too, as the enzymatic system's action is enhanced, better utilising insulin.

The fact that aerobic exercise is continuous exertion for an hour or more each day makes it especially important physiologically. As your muscles are worked, waste products, especially lactic acid, build up. As the exercising continues, these products are gently released. Warmdown stretching completes the action. Repeated exercise sessions increase the ability of the venous system to cope with excess waste.

In addition, aerobics make you more alert, more energetic and, therefore, more productive at work. The more oxygen circulating through the body, the more oxygen reaches the brain, stimulating the firing of neurons over the synapses, the electric charge that produces 'thought'. This 'speeding' effect is much the same as that produced by caffeine or artificial 'uppers', but it is pure and organic and therefore has no harmful side-effects. Your revived and strengthened body is more attractive, more appealing. You feel better – alive, supple, beautiful.

But what about those bulges in your mid-riff and along your hips, swinging like saddlebags? Can aerobics get rid of these? Of course. But an even quicker method involves spot-toning in combination with aerobic work. Spot-toning concentrates on individual muscle groups, isolating them and forcing them to work extra hard. My routine of specific 'isometric' exercises, as they are called, will aid greatly in slimming your thighs and waist and flattening your stomach.

But before starting the exercises, you must understand that you are not merely dealing with three areas of the body. You are working innumerable muscles, tendons and ligaments. At the end of each exercise in the routine is a list of the specific muscles used. By referring to the diagram of the muscles, you can understand where your power to extend or flex a particular limb comes from. In exercising, therefore, you can concentrate on the correct muscles, in isolation, to tone the parts of your body that need it most.

All the muscles referred to in the exercises are skeletal muscles and function to move parts of the skeleton with attachments across joints called tendons. They are arranged in opposed pairs, one on either side of the bone, and control movement on leverage principles. A contraction shortens the muscle and flexes the joint; a stretch extends the joint.

Additional muscles are involved to steady and support the action. All these are voluntary muscles; therefore they act on brain impulses which, in turn, are the reactions of sensations from the muscles. Everything works on mirror principles, a confidence game learned by instinct.

The tissue of skeletal muscles is made up of protein (20%), minerals (5%) and water (75%). Thus it is essential to take in plenty of fluids, proteins and nutrients – vitamins and minerals – to keep your muscles in peak condition.

Structurally, the muscles are made up of short fibres held together in bundles which narrow down to fibrous tissue, the tendon. It is important to realise that this tendon is not elastic like the muscle. The elasticity of the muscle itself is determined by its warmth. A cold muscle is brittle and hard, it does not 'give', and this puts extra strain on the tendon. Therefore, especially in areas of the body where the tendon is long, like the calves, you must keep the stretchy muscles in good condition. A broken tendon is a very painful injury which involves complex

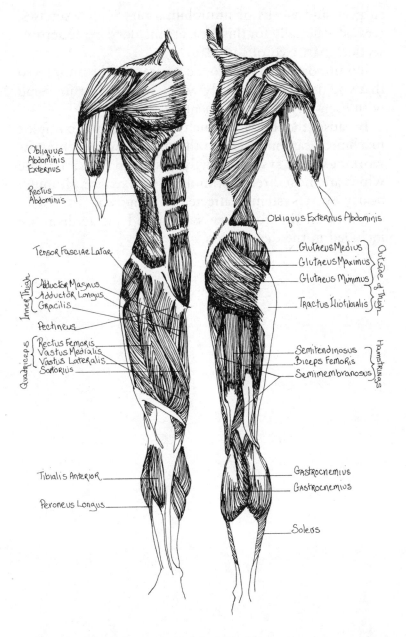

An anterior and posterior view of the body showing the various muscles.

13

surgery and weeks of immobilisation. Some exercises, created especially for this area, are included in the aerobic section (part two of my plan).

It is important to refer to the diagram of the muscles so that you understand exactly which muscle you are using with each physical movement.

Because the body is such an incredibly complex machine, I can only scratch the surface in explaining its workings. The systems briefly described here are those which are most directly stimulated by exercise, although nearly every system is affected in some way.

Notes on the gustatory system and metabolism are included in the diet section.

Exercise benefits the mind. As mentioned earlier, the sense of control over your body makes you feel powerful and well-ordered. This promotes relaxation and peace of mind, which in turn suppresses unpleasant emotions, such as hostility, anger, jealousy, depression and frustration, as well as physical problems such as insomnia, fatigue, overeating and impotency. In fact, exercise is so positive, that an example can be found of nearly every psychological benefit imaginable.

However, it is essential to get your mind in shape *before* you attempt to get your body in shape. A programme, no matter how carefully put together, planned and followed, is a waste of time unless it is accompanied by a change of attitude. You cannot wish yourself thin, but you can *think* yourself thin. In fact, I believe this mental change is as important as sticking to the exercises, and if all this book does is to give you a better outlook on the world of fitness, then I feel it has gone a long way to achieving its ends.

But remember, slimming those flabby areas of your body through exercise is not a life-or-death project. It is meant to be an enjoyable, positive experience. Do not become obsessed with the idea of being thin.

Many young girls are influenced by glossy magazines which put forward the idea that the near-starvation look is desirable. This causes many to diet well below their natural weight, jeopardising both their health and their looks.

Thinness will not solve all your problems. It is not the secret to success nor to gaining compliments. It is only

15

the self-confidence you achieve by successfully shaping your figure, that can change your life in these ways. Remember, be happy while slimming to ensure happiness when slim. You do not want to look like a girl in a magazine. Your goal is to look like you. And like it.

Of course it is difficult, if not impossible, not to be influenced by the current cultural pressure to diet, diet, diet. Only the anorexic personality succumbs completely, however. You can use the pressure positively by starting a weight-loss programme like mine. Just be sure you have read the appropriate commentary fully and know what you are doing.

Once you have decided to follow my diet and exercise programme, stick to it. Discipline and concentration are all-important to achieve results. You must exercise regularly. Not only because this will improve your body tone and aerobic capacity, but as an important safety precaution. If you exercise vigorously only once in a while, you will cause more harm to your body than good. Your heart will not have been sufficiently strengthened; you could even bring on a heart attack.

You should exercise every day for no less than half an hour. If this is not possible, try to do so at least four times a week.

Do not start tomorrow, start exercising today! Don't put off beginning your exercise programme until a less hectic future date. You will never get around to it if you do. Fit the programme into your life now, and soon it will become as urgent as those other responsibilities.

Clothing
You should wear clothes that you reserve specially for your exercise sessions. Anything non-restricting and comfortable will do. Shorts or tracksuit and a sweatshirt are fine for both the exercise routine and aerobic activity.

Or why not wear something colourful and fun – like a jazzy leotard and tights!

Environment
Choose a warm (or cool in hot weather), pleasant environment for your routine. Set up a specific area that has plenty of space for swings and kicks. If possible, exercise in front of a large mirror. Watching yourself helps you to perform exercises properly. If you do not have a large mirror, try a window or a sliding glass door, which will give a good reflection, especially at night. Or work in front of a complicated poster or painting – this will give you something interesting to contemplate.

Equipment
Music is absolutely essential. For indoor exercises, tapes are preferable to records as vigorous activity may cause the needle to jump. A portable stereo, such as the popular 'Sony Walkman', is ideal for the jogger.

Choose tunes with a fast, steady beat. These should be songs you enjoy, light rather than melodramatic. Disco, new wave and 60's rock and roll are good choices.

Use a small foam rubber pad or towel for floor exercises.

Elimination of Distractions
Choose a time of day when you are least likely to be interrupted. Take the phone off the hook. Do not answer the door bell. Do not try to cook or monitor the washing during your exercise time. This is the one moment of the day when you can afford to be selfish.

Do's and Don'ts
1. *Do* check with your doctor before beginning any exercise routine that you have never tried before. He

will give you the signal to go ahead as he knows you, your body and your capacity to perform specific exercises.

2. *Don't* eat heavy meals at least two hours before vigorous exercise. This can cause cramp and nausea. Working on an empty stomach has no ill-effects.

3. *Don't* drink ice-cold drinks after exercise so as to avoid irritating the heart's rhythm. But *do* drink something, in order to replace fluids lost via sweating as you do not want to become dehydrated.

4. *Do* focus your goals. Write down waist, thigh and stomach measurements desired plus trouser and skirt size. Also note down your current sizes and measurements. Pin a note to your wall as a reminder.

The Three-Part Plan

ONE: THE EXERCISES

I have divided the exercises into twelve parts. Each part works on a particular muscle or set of muscles as indicated and follows a specific sequence. A point-by-point explanation of each movement is accompanied by photographs showing exactly how certain positions are achieved. Not every point is illustrated, so the text must be studied carefully before you begin. Each exercise must be completed in full to obtain maximum stretch and tone benefit.

The routine should take between 30 and 45 minutes depending upon your fitness and familiarity with the movements. Before embarking upon the exercises, make sure you have read my introductory chapters, as the results you achieve will be in direct proportion to your understanding of your body.

At the back of the book, on pages 74–79, are charts indicating the number of times you are to repeat each exercise throughout the thirty-day programme. Refer to these each day before you begin. The cue to repeat muscular motion is the word '*Repeat*' at certain points in the exercise. When you reach a '*Repeat*', stop, refer to the chart for that day and repeat what has come just before in the sequence as many times as is suggested.

The charts are divided into three categories according to the level of pre-routine fitness. The NOVICE is those of you who are unfamiliar with a regular exercise programme. Maybe you are new to the world of fitness, or perhaps you used to do a particular sport but have just let yourself go. Whatever your circumstances, the NOVICE routine is designed for the beginner. It is advisable for

19

everyone with any doubts about their fitness to begin at this level. If, after a week or two, you find the routine sequences too short, you may step up to a more difficult level. Moving up is preferable to moving down.

The KEEN participants are those of you who are mentally in excellent shape to perform exercises. Your body is much more attuned to physical strain than the NOVICE, but still needs to be shaped properly before it can work at the advanced level. You will approach the programme energetically, finding it a definite challenge.

The EXPERT is the advanced participant. You are probably already an exercise addict, but if not, you at least have the physical potential to be one. The exercise repetitions at this level have been geared to make you work hard. You will be pushing yourself progressively and patiently, firming specific muscles. Keeping fit requires adherence to a regular schedule, as does getting fit.

This exercise routine is for both men and women. A male beginner, however, may need to go straight to the KEEN level as his muscles, for hormonal reasons, are generally stronger than a woman's and therefore he can take more strain right from the start.

The 'point of no return' is a term I have used to describe that delicate point of tension where the muscle is pushed to its limit. This point is reached before definite pain occurs; it might be accompanied by a 'glowing' sensation which Jane Fonda calls 'the burn'. Do not push further than this point, as you can cause damage, but try to hold the muscle there for several seconds. Next time, your 'point of no return' may be farther. Remember, too, *never* bounce into a stretch. Control the push, as well as the release, into a flex or contraction.

Breathing is very important when performing these exercises. Never hold your breath, but concentrate on exhaling rather than inhaling. This will ensure that oxygen fills the lungs to their maximum capacity. Exhale as you exert your muscles: when you bend, pull or push. Inhale as you lower and release. This brings extra oxygen to the muscles when they need it most. It also reduces the risk of stomach cramps. Breathing in this way may take a little getting used to, as we normally breathe in reverse, but concentrate and in time it will become natural.

Having studied the exercises and prepared yourself properly by following my guidelines, you are ready to begin. Good luck!

Starting position

It is important to begin the routine in the correct position and to maintain this position throughout unless otherwise advised.

Stand up straight, legs shoulder-width apart and relaxed. Shoulders should be level and loose, neither hunched nor lifted. Stomach must be pulled in and pelvis tilted under; buttocks tight. Try to concentrate on making movements graceful and fluid.

Warm-up (*the same for all levels*)
This is a necessary appetiser for the stomach, waist and thigh routine. It is important to loosen *all over* first.

Neck Rolls
Neck exercises release the tension in the neck and shoulders which has built up after a long day at work. They also wake up sleepy stiff joints in the early morning.

Start with 10 nods to the left, then 10 to the right, 10 forward and 10 back. Roll the head in a full circle 3 times, first to the left, then to the right. Reverse and *repeat*.

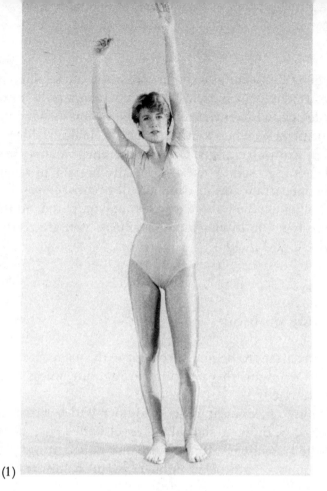

(1)

Stretch Ups
To continue loosening up, stretch your arms straight above your head. Pull both of them upwards at the same time as if you were trying to touch the sky. *Repeat* 5 times. Then alternate arms, pulling one up and then the other. *Repeat* (1).

Waist Reaches
Without dropping out of time with your music, pull your torso to the side from the waist up, stretching out both arms (2). Feel the stretch in your waist. Alternate sides and *repeat*.

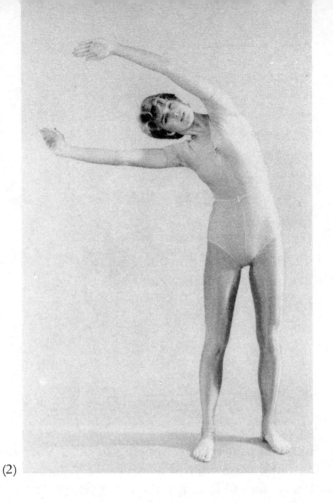

(2)

Hamstring Stretch
1. Bring your legs together and resume starting position. Bend forward with your arms stretched straight out to the sides. Your legs should remain straight. Bend all the way until your upper body forms an 'L' with your legs.
2. Now inch your back down in controlled stretches. Feel the pull on the back of your knees. Inch for 5 counts.
3. Lean the top of your body all the way to the floor, keeping your legs straight. Grip the front of your

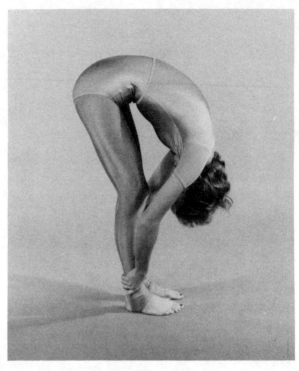

(3)

ankles and pull down, striving to 'kiss' your knees (3). Hold for 5 counts.
4. Release the ankle grip and relax in this position. Feel the hamstrings ease into a lengthened stretch. Inhale. Exhale.
5. Grip your ankles again and pull down 5 times.

More Hamstring Stretches
1. Bend your knees slightly and place your hands flat on the floor about eight inches directly in front of your feet. Legs remain shoulder-width apart. Make sure your feet remain flat also.
2. Straighten your knees, keeping hands on floor.
3. Bend your knees again, performing the stretch in one fast, smooth motion. *Repeat* 10 times.

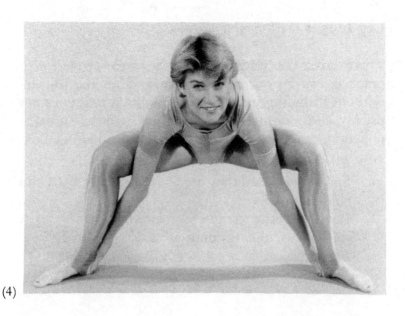

(4)

Frog Stretch

1. Walk your hands back to your ankles and straighten your legs. Keep your feet flat on the floor. Memorise the pull on hamstrings. Place your hands around the back of the ankles from the inside.
2. Lower body, buttocks first, until you reach a full squat (4). No giggles, this is the best way to stretch your inner thighs. Hold for 8 counts.
3. Lift buttocks and try to straighten your legs. Lower. Lift and lower for a controlled count of 5.

To finish warm-up, release grip on your ankles and straighten your knees. Arms should dangle in front of you. Let your back relax for a few seconds. Then slowly begin to roll up, vertebra by vertebra. Beware of straightening too fast or you will become dizzy. Make sure your legs are not locked. When you are completely upright resume starting position. Smile! You are now ready to work out.

25

Leg lunges (*for trimming thighs*)

This exercise is a continuation of the warm-up and, with practice, can be started immediately after the roll-up, without throwing your music. The disco beat does not usually allow hesitation! Always try to keep stomach pulled in, pelvis under and back straight. Do not hold your breath.

1. Spread legs until they are about two feet apart and straighten knees.
2. Reach left hand to right foot, letting right arm reach up behind, and bending at waist (5). Straighten. *Repeat.*

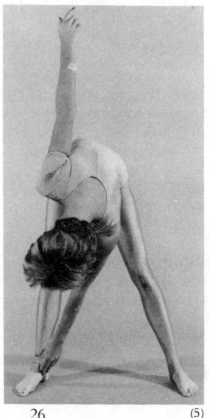 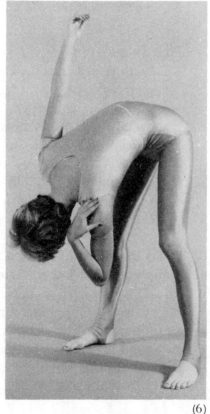

(5)

(6)

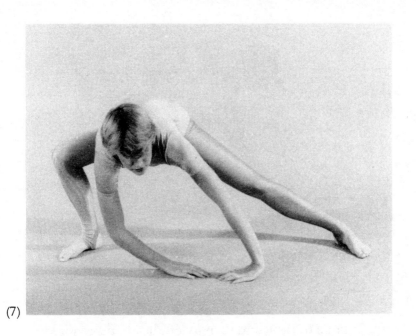

(7)

3. Reverse the motion by touching the left foot with the right hand. *Repeat.*

4. Next, place the left fist on shoulder, elbow straight in front of you. Bend over and attempt to touch your elbow to your right foot (6). At the same time, bend right leg so that body is in semi-lunge position. Feel a strong pull along the back of the right thigh and inner left leg. Straighten, lunge again and *repeat.*

5. Reverse to opposite motion and *repeat.*

6. After these repetitions have been completed, place hands on floor in front of you.

7. Lunge right leg to side and bend right elbow as far as possible. Strive to place right elbow on floor (7), but do not force yourself lest you run the risk of injury. Hold position and then straighten. *Repeat.*

8. Now, from the position just assumed, straighten arms. Hold out to sides at shoulder level.

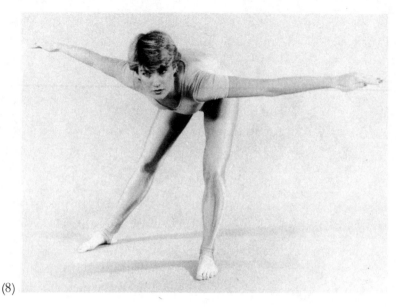

(8)

9.   Lunge to right and then to left, head up and looking ahead (8). Is that a fly on the wall? Stretch forward to see. Touch chest to top of thigh with each lunge. *Repeat.*

10. Straighten torso and lunge from side to side with back upright. *Repeat.*

Muscles used: Quadriceps, gracilis, adductors, tensor fasciae latae, tractus iliotbialis, gastrocnemius.

Waist pulls and twists *(for slimming waist)*

Remember to pull directly to the side. Neither the upper body nor the hips should lean backwards or forwards. Pretend that you are doing this exercise between two cacti. A lean either way will thus have drastic consequences – that is, no trim waist! Also, make sure you complete *all* the pulls to one side without stopping *before* starting pulls on the opposite side.

28

1. Assume starting position, legs relaxed. With hands on hips, lean upper torso directly to the right side from the waist. Feel the pull along the left side of the body.
2. Straighten all the way up, then lean again. *Repeat* movements should be complete and precise. Concentrate on the straightening up motion and try and pull down a fraction further each time.
3. Now drop the right arm and raise the left arm above head (9). Pull down and up again. *Repeat*.
4. Bring hands together above head and pull to side with straight arms (10). Straighten and *repeat*.

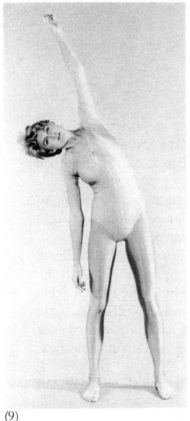

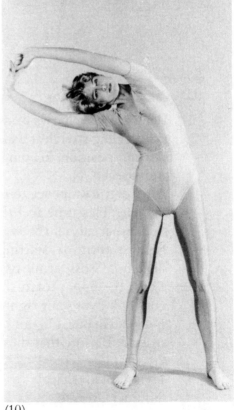

(9) (10)

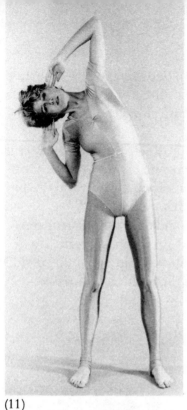 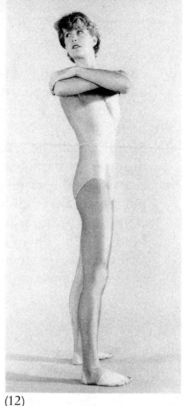

(11)   (12)

5. Bend arms at elbows bringing hands to ears. Pull to side, feeling stretch at waist (11). Straighten body to starting position, keeping arms at ears! Bend again and *repeat*.

6. After entire sequence to the right, *repeat*, pulling to the left. This time feel the stretch along the right side, especially in the waist area.

7. Now return to starting position. Bend knees slightly. Cross arms over chest at elbow level. Twist the upper torso sharply to the right so that you look over your right shoulder (12). Turn torso and head in one. Do not twist hips nor wrench neck around. Be sure that these areas remain stationary. *Repeat*.

8. Twist torso sharply to left and look over left shoulder. *Repeat*.

9. Next open arms wide and twist to right. *Repeat,* then twist to left.
10. Alternate swings from left to right.

Variations: Pull left arm up with elbow bent as you bend in the opposite direction. The right arm should stretch to the side also. Straighten and stretch. *Repeat.* Switch to opposite side and *repeat.*

Muscles used: Internal and external obliques, transverse.

Leg lifts *(for trimming thighs)*

These thigh isometrics have been specially designed for maximum trimming results. Remember never to touch foot to floor between repetitions; keep it at least three inches off the floor. Control movement on the way *down* as well as on the way up. Keep leg straight. Make the movements complete and graceful. Do not cheat by merely lifting halfway.

1. Starting position for these exercises is on the floor. Lie down on the right side. Left leg should be directly on top of the right one, although the right can be slightly bent for support. It is important to keep the torso from rolling forward. Use the right arm as support for upper body, holding it in a 90° angle to side. Do not sink down into the shoulder. Once you have achieved this position, feel comfortable and graceful. You are ready to begin!
2. Raise the left leg straight up. Keep the knee straight and point the toe. Lift until the leg is at a 45° angle to the body (13). Hold and lower with control. Feel the quadriceps and inner thigh muscles working. *Repeat.*
3. Next raise the same leg to the same angle with the foot flexed (14). *Repeat.*

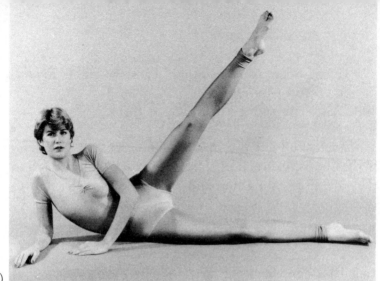

(13)

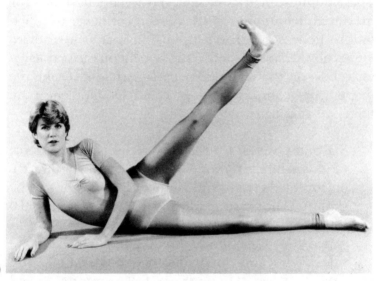

(14)

4. After the last repetition, kick the leg straight forward in front of you. Keep it stiff but make sure the foot remains flexed (15). Bring it back to the starting position without touching the floor and kick again. Do not move hips or torso. *Repeat.*

5. With foot kicked in front of you as far as it can go with leg straight, lift up the leg. Foot should be

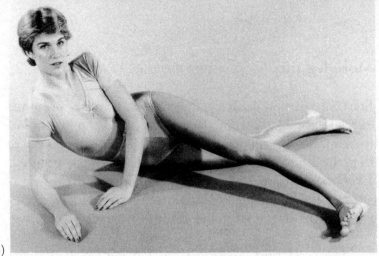

(15)

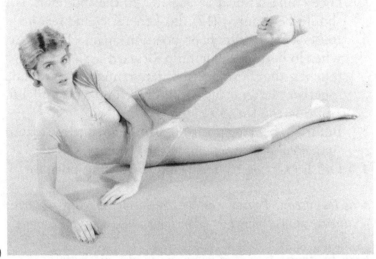

(16)

flexed. Lift all the way to the 'point of no return' – the point where you feel a definite 'glow'. (16). The buttocks should be squeezed tight. Lower leg to three inches off floor and raise again. *Repeat.* Then return to starting position.

6. *Repeat* entire sequence with right leg.

Muscles used: *Tensor fasciae latae, gluteus minimus, gluteus maximus, pectineus.*

More leg lifts (*for trimming thighs and buttocks*)

Starting position is on the floor once again: see previous exercise for instruction. Remember to keep all movements fluid. On roll leg lifts (instructions 2–3), make sure that the lifted leg is kept straight and the toe pointed. Every other day begin the entire sequence with the opposite leg. Be sure to release hips after these leg lift exercises with warm-down stretches found on pages 51–54.

1. From starting position bend left leg up so that the knee comes as near as possible to the shoulder. Toe should be pointed (17). Lower, raise, and *repeat*.
2. Raise left leg into bent position again (18). Now, when lowering, roll left hip forward so that it almost touches the floor. Arms can come forward and together. Extend leg straight behind you and lift, pointing the toe (19).
3. Return to bent leg position. Roll again into leg extension. *Repeat* as one, single movement.
4. Finish exercise by returning to starting position.

Muscles used: *Tensor fasciae, adductor magnus, gracilis pectineus, gluteal muscles, adductor brevis, adductor longus*.

Fire hydrant lifts (*for trimming thighs and buttocks*)

These have often been called the 'dog' exercises for obvious reasons. Here is your chance to lift your leg and pay back that beagle who gets so desperate in the park!

Remember not to lower leg to floor during repetition or between series of repetitions. Always keep it at least three inches from floor. Be sure you perform a suitable warm-down exercise after this thigh and buttock workout. A good one is the 'Mecca' pose, found on page 40.

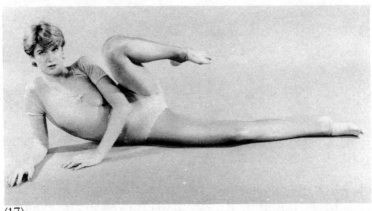

(17)

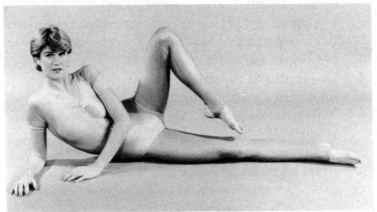

(18)

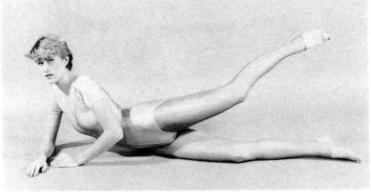

(19)

35

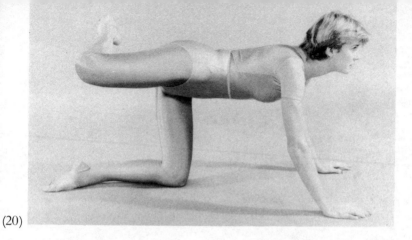

(20)

1. Starting position is on the hands and knees. The back should be flat, stomach tucked in and weight evenly distributed.
2. Lift right leg, keeping knee bent to the side until the thigh is parallel to the floor. This should be about hip height (20).
3. Lower almost to starting position but do not touch floor. Lift again and *repeat*.
4. Now lift right leg and extend it to the side, opening at knee (21).
5. Bend, straighten and *repeat*.
6. Bring right leg in and under you. Tuck knee into chest, bringing forehead down to meet (22).

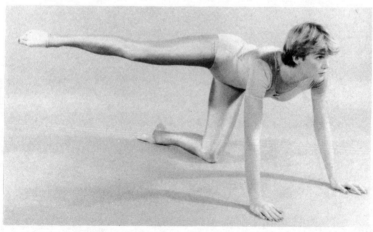

(21)

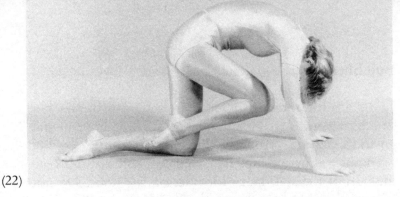

(22)

7. Extend right leg behind, keeping it straight and toe pointed. Lift as high as possible (23). Feel definite stretch in buttock and thigh.

8. Lower leg and bring it and forehead together again (22). Lift again and *repeat* stretch.

9. After last repetition, keep right leg extended. Lift it behind and up a few inches. Lower, keeping leg straight, toe pointed. Lift and *repeat*.

10. *Repeat* entire sequence of exercises using opposite leg.

Muscles used: Hamstrings, gluteal muscles.

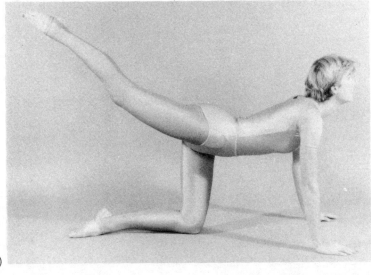

(23)

Bun burners *(for toning buttocks, trimming thighs and hips)*

These are the most difficult exercises in the series but should nevertheless be approached with dedication and gusto. They are primarily done to tone buttocks, but work the thighs and hips also. Remember to try and keep the heel of the stationary foot flat on the floor. Do not worry when blood rushes to the head. It is simply bringing more oxygen to the brain, a condition that does more good than harm. The body spends most of its time working against gravity to supply the upper body with blood, so a little physical help now and then is certainly beneficial.

Try to keep palms flat. Putting your entire weight on your fingers will only cause pain. Do not lower leg to floor between repetitions or series of repetitions. Be sure you perform a brief warm–down, such as the 'Mecca' on page 40, before continuing the programme.

1. Starting position for these exercises is leaning forward with feet on floor, legs straight, heels down.

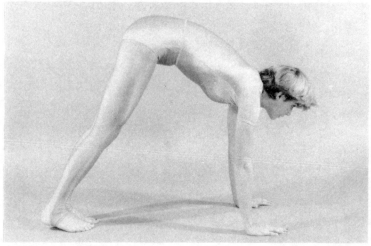

(24)

38

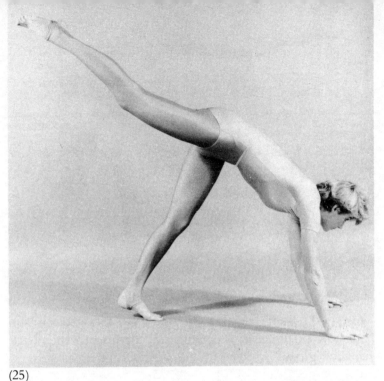

(25)

Hands should touch floor about two feet from toes (24). The body should be in an upside-down 'V' and remain so throughout the exercise.

2. From here, lift the right leg straight up behind you. Point the toe and make sure the knee is straight. Lift to the 'point of no return', feeling the stretch in the buttocks (25). Lower, but not to floor, and *repeat*.

3. Lift right leg to a position parallel with the buttocks. Swing to side until leg is perpendicular to the torso. Keep leg straight and flex foot (26).

4. Return right leg to position straight behind (25). Swing forward again and *repeat*.

Variations: For those particularly keen on working the buttocks, this exercise can be supplemented with variation on the 'FIRE HYDRANT' exercises (page 34). Bring the bent knee in to touch the chest and then extend it behind, lifting high, toe pointed. Bend

39

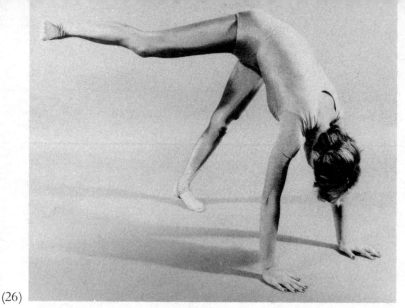

(26)

again and *repeat*. Try all four 'FIRE HYDRANT' exercises in this new position in repetitions according to the chart. Feel the glow!

Muscles used: Gluteus maximus, gluteus minimus, gluteus medius; hamstrings; semitendinosus, biceps femoris, semimembranosus.

Warm-down interval: *the Mecca pose*

The 'Mecca' pose is an excellent exercise to relax the buttocks, leg and back muscles. The spine is eased, too, in this position.

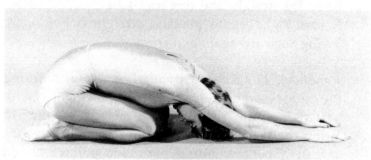

(27)

Kneel on floor. Lean upper body over the legs. Extend the arms out in front of you as far as they will go and place hands on floor. Walk arms out a few inches further with fingers if possible (27). Now, allow entire body to relax and rest in this position. Hold for 5 counts. Walk arms out further. Feel the loosening in the buttocks. Hold for another 5 counts. Inhale. Exhale. Sit up and get ready to begin the second half of the wonderful routine!

Open leg stretches *(for trimming thighs and slimming waist)*

Make sure the back is straight throughout these stretches. Do not bring body forward to increase the stretch in the thighs as this only tenses the shoulders and decreases the pull in the legs. It will take a while to be able to sit up comfortably. You are now reversing all the damage done from years spent hunching over school desks in improperly designed chairs. You cannot undo in a day what has taken many years to develop. Be patient; results will be slow, but definite.

1. The starting position for these stretches is sitting on floor, legs spread, with both thighs and calves pressed down and knees straight. Sit up with back straight and torso lifted. Arms should be resting on hips. There should be an expanse of muscle and tissue between the ribcage and the pelvic bones. This cavity is revealed by lifting the back through.
2. Lift the right leg 4 inches off the floor (28). Hold for 5 seconds. Release slowly. *Repeat*.
3. Lift left leg. Hold for 5 seconds. Release and *repeat*.
4. Now lift both legs up together and hold. Bring them together in front of you in lifted position. Open again and *repeat*.

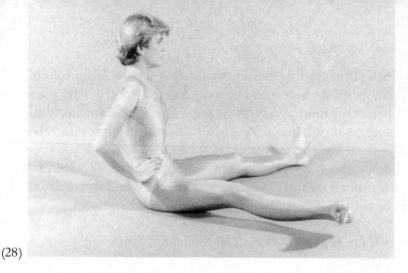

(28)

5. Next reach arms up towards ears with bent elbows. Bend at waist towards the right, keeping both shoulders facing forward (29).
6. Raise body to starting position. *Repeat* bending movement.
7. After repetition, *repeat* entire sequence to the left.

Muscles used: Gracilus and adductors on the leg lifts; obliques and adductors on the side pulls.

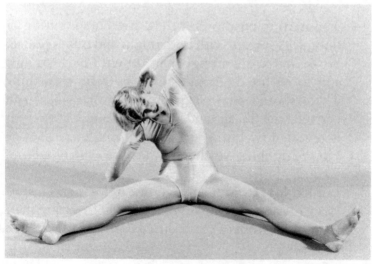

(29)

Stomach strengthening sequence *(for flattening stomach and slimming waist)*

Remember to keep stomach pulled in tight and back straight.

1. Sit up straight, facing forward with legs together in front of you, knees bent. Place hands behind head with elbows out to the side.
2. Lean back until the upper body is at a 45° angle to the floor.
3. Twist torso to the right, pivoting at the waist (30). Return to centre position. *Repeat.*
4. Twist torso to the left, then return to centre. *Repeat.*
5. Bend to right again, this time placing the elbow outside the right knee. This involves a slight lean to the side (31).

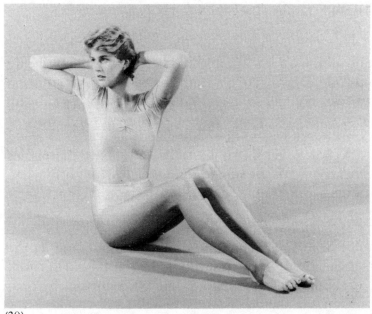

(30)

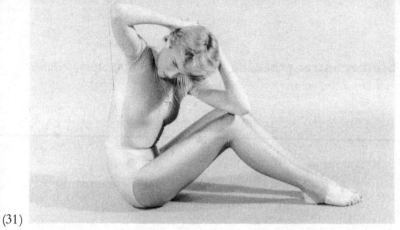

6. Return to centre and repeat movement towards the right.
7. At end of repetition, *repeat* bending exercise to the left.

Muscles used: Rectus abdominus, internal and external obliques, transverse, erector spinae.

Sit-ups *(for flattening stomach and slimming waist)*

Feet should always remain flat on the floor during sit-ups. If you cannot complete the exercise without lifting up your feet, you are not ready for sit-ups. Your stomach muscles are still too weak. They need to be gradually strengthened by concentrating on curl-ups and -downs. Omit the sit-ups until you are ready.

Do not forget that it is *vital* that the stomach muscles do *all* the work. Be sure to round the back slightly when lifting, too; a straight back leads to reliance on hip flexors.

1. Lie flat on your back with knees bent, legs relaxed. Place hands behind head (32). Look up and let the weight of head rest in cradled hands. The neck should be relaxed. Locate stomach muscles by contracting them.

44

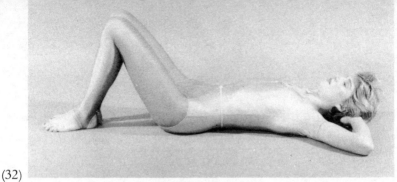

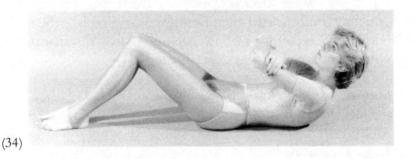

(34)

2. Lift upper torso until it is at a 45° angle to the floor (33). Do not go into a full sit-up yet. Feel abdominal muscles contract.
3. Lower and *repeat*.
4. Raise body to a sitting position. Hands should come forward and cross over chest. Lower body to the same 45° angle (34). This is a curl-down, the exact opposite of the curling-up exercise you have just completed.

45

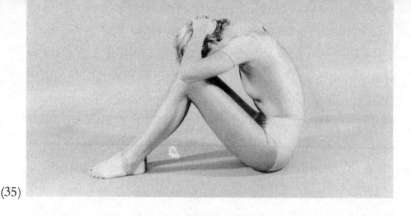

(35)

5. Raise torso to sitting position. Lower and *repeat*.
6. Lie down on floor again. Head should remain cradled in hands. Now raise body all the way up to the knees in a full sit-up. (35). Make sure that you are using contracted stomach muscles to lift.
7. Slowly release stomach and lower body back to the floor. *Repeat*.

Variations: When stomach muscles are strong enough, you may omit the curl-ups and -downs and replace them with extra repetitions of the sit-ups. Also, try sit-ups with legs extended, but don't lift legs!

Muscles used: *Rectus abdominus, internal and external obliques, transverse.*

Leg extensions (*for flattening stomach and slimming waist*)

Breathe out during stomach muscle contraction so that you do not burst the peritoneum. Do not use your neck to pull up torso! Also, if you feel a strain in the trapezius region, you are doing the exercise wrong. Stop, look up and let your head fall back, relaxed. Feel the muscles in the stomach contract and work. A rather nauseous feeling sometimes accompanies these exercises, especially if the muscles are weak. Do not panic about this. You are unlikely to vomit as a result. Perseverance will strengthen

46

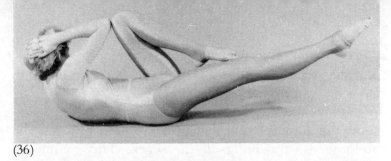

(36)

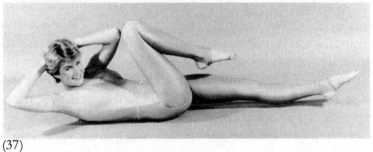

(37)

the abdominals and soon you will be able to perform the entire sequence without pain or nausea.

1. Lie down flat on your back on the floor. Arms should be relaxed at the sides.
2. Extend right leg out, toe pointed. The foot should be raised a few inches off the floor.
3. Bend the left knee in towards the chest. At the same time touch the left knee with the right elbow. (36).
4. Reverse movement by extending left leg while you bend in right knee. Touch right knee with the left elbow (37). *Repeat*. (This exercise should be performed quickly and fluidly. You should not, however, circle legs in a 'bicycle' motion. Concentrate on extending one leg straight in front of you with the toe pointed towards the wall and then bending it in with the calf parallel to the floor.)
5. *Repeat* sequence with foot flexed.

Muscles used: *Rectus abdominus, internal and external obliques, transverse.*

Raised leg sequence *(for flattening stomach, slimming waist, trimming thighs and buttocks)*

Once again, make sure that your stomach muscles, the abdominals, are doing *all* the work. This cannot be emphasised enough. The tendency is to use the shoulders or, even more cunningly, the hip flexors. These are the muscles which run down from the spine and divide off to attach to the head of each thigh bone. These are usually strong muscles because you use them to walk. You cannot actually see the flexor muscles working, so cheating is easy. If you feel a pull in the back, compensate by contracting the stomach and allowing it to 'take over'. Follow the exercise as carefully outlined here and you will perform properly. You do not want to overstretch the stomach muscles because this can make a 'bulge' worse.

1. Lie down flat on your back with legs stretched straight out forward. Hands are clasped behind the head with the face towards the sky. Lift both legs using the stomach muscles. Keep legs straight. Lift until they are perpendicular to the body (38).

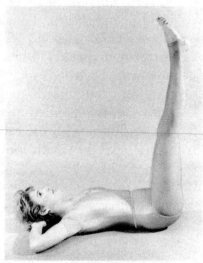

(38)

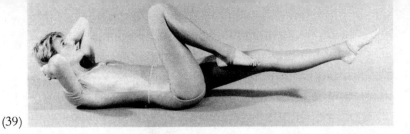

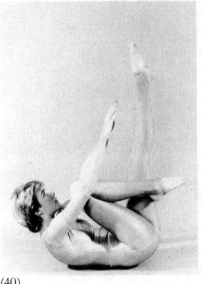

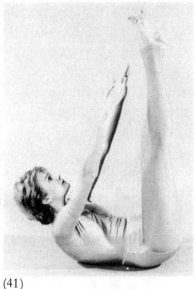

(39)

(40)

(41)

2. Keeping legs straight, lower a few inches. Then raise again. *Repeat.*

3. Bend the right knee toward you while holding the left leg a few inches off the ground (39).

4. Lift top half of body off the floor a few inches and extend the arms. Strive to touch the toes with the fingers. Concentrate on making controlled, complete stretches (40). *Repeat.* Switch legs and *repeat.*

5. Lift both legs up together at a 90° angle to the body. Reach up with arms and hands and strive to touch toes (41). Be sure you are lifting with the abdominal muscles, *not* the shoulders. *Repeat.*

Muscles used: Rectus abdominus, internal and external obliques, transverse, quadriceps, gluteal muscles.

49

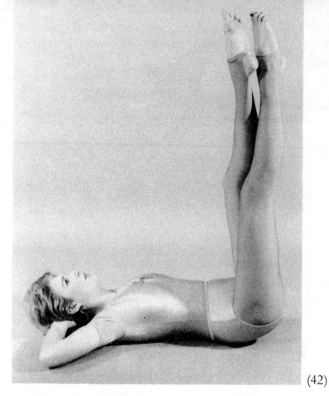

(42)

Scissors *(for flattening stomach and trimming thighs)*

Always use the stomach muscles while raising and lowering. Your back should not arch at any time.

1. Lie flat on your back on the floor. Raise both legs together into perpendicular position. Scissor them left to right. Toes should be pointed (42). *Repeat.*

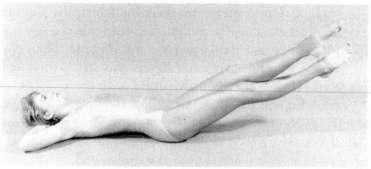

(43)

2. Continue scissors up and down as if walking with small steps. Flex feet.
3. Lower legs until they are 6 inches off the floor and scissor kick them left to right again, with toes pointed (43).
4. Finally, scissor legs up and down, feet flexed. *Repeat.*
5. Release abdominals by pulling knees into chest tightly and holding for 5–10 seconds.

Muscles used: *Rectus abdominus, internal and external obliques, hamstrings.*

Warm-down (*the same for all levels*)

The warm-down is just as important as the warm-up, if not *more* important. The muscles in the hips, waist, stomach, thighs and even the calves have become tensed through continual contraction. A release is needed to stretch the muscles back out and to restore the balance of acids in the fibres. By neglecting to warm down a muscle, you run a higher risk of having stiff and sore muscles the next day. The first two exercises, the 'hip and hamstring release' (pictures 44 and 45) should always be performed after the leg lifts and before going on with the rest of the routine.

Hip and Hamstring Release
1. Begin by lying flat on your back, arms relaxed at your sides. Take a deep breath. Hold and exhale, feeling the body relax.
2. Bend the right knee and pull it, with your arms, towards your chest. Hold for 5 seconds feeling the hip flexors release (44).
3. Grab the right heel with the left hand and grab the

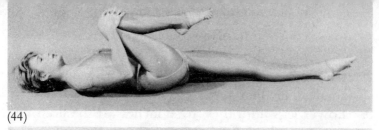

(44)

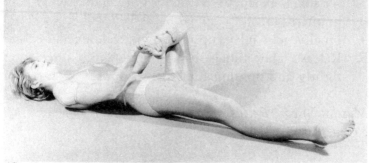

(45)

right ankle with the right hand. Pull foot and calf towards you. Be sure you pull leg and foot together as merely pulling at the foot will only twist the ankle. The knee should rotate to the right (45).

4. Concentrate on pushing your knee down. Unless you are super flexible, the knee will come nowhere near the floor and it is important that you do not try to force it. Just push until you feel the contracted buttock and hip muscles crack and release. Hold for 5 seconds.

5. Return leg to starting position. *Repeat* entire sequences with left leg.

The Killer Stretch

1. Sit up, keeping legs straight and together in front of you.

2. Grab toes and flex feet hard, so that the heels are lifted off the floor.

3. Now pull the top of body down over the legs, keeping the heels lifted off the floor. Continue reaching, concentrating on touching the elbows to floor. Hold for 5 seconds and release. *Repeat*.

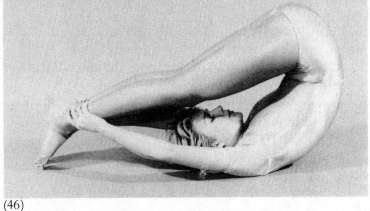

(46)

The Plough
1. From the lying down position, pull knees into chest.
2. Lift hips up, bend knees over head.
3. Extend legs straight out and together. Touch pointed toes to the floor behind your head (46). Hold.
4. Drop knees to either side of head, next to the ears. Relax spine and roll slightly. Hold.
5. Come out of position by unfolding legs first and then rolling body down vertebra by vertebra. Legs should remain straight until they touch the floor in front of you.

The Frog
1. Lie on your back with legs bent.

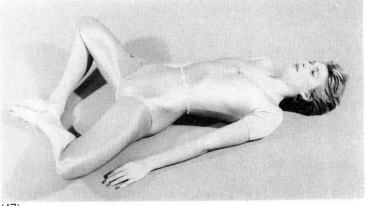

(47)

2. Draw the legs outward, bringing the soles of the feet together as they extend.
3. Lower thighs and knees as close to the floor as possible (47).
4. Hold for 10 seconds.

Final warm-down

Repeat the warm-up sequence (on pages 21–25) in reverse, starting with the 'frog stretch' and ending with the 'head rolls' to the right and then to the left. You should be able to stretch and bend much further, bounce much higher, reach much further.

Congratulations! You are now on your way towards a healthier, trimmer, more attractive body. And don't you feel *good*?

TWO: THE AEROBICS ROUTINE

An important complement to the exercise routine is an aerobic activity, seriously undertaken each day. Any form of exercise that makes your body work hard, demanding extra oxygen, is 'aerobian'. You must now decide what type of aerobic exercise you are to follow. Being a true Californian, I tend to urge everyone to try jogging. Running or jogging (the terms are interchangeable) is, I think, the most enjoyable and effective form of physical exercise. It is safe, simple and convenient. It requires minimum preparation and time and can be done at any time, anywhere.

However, if you are not keen on jogging, there are many other forms of aerobian exercise that are just as beneficial: dancing, cycling, jumping, swimming, even walking briskly, are all excellent. Race-walking has currently captured a lot of attention on the east coast of the United States as an alternative to jogging. This is a sequence of brisk steps executed in such a way that contact with the ground is never broken.

Whatever form of aerobic exercise you choose, be sure you prepare properly beforehand. Pay particular attention to the following:

1. If you are completely new to aerobic exercise, consult your doctor before embarking on any programme. But I can guarantee that, except in unusual circumstances, he will encourage you to participate.
2. Before each individual routine, be sure to warm up with a good stretch. It is especially important to stretch the hamstrings, calves and Achilles tendon. I

have included some exercises for you to follow on pages 62–63.

3. Do not try to do too much too soon. Listen to your body. Learn the difference between destructive and constructive pain. A 'glowing' sensation is good and indicates positive dangers, while a sharp tug or persistent ache signals potential damage.

4. Beware of aerobic indigestion. Always stop with the feeling that you could have gone on a bit longer. This will help you get up (often in the dark of the early morning) and go the next day. If you do more than you can handle, you might become fed up with the whole thing.

5. Make your programme regular, every day if you can. Four times a week at the very least. Anything less than this is token exercise and really will not cause significant body changes. But do not feel guilty if you miss your daily quota now and then. Just push yourself a little bit harder the next time!

6. Do not compete with anyone except yourself. Play only against a flabby, out-of-shape body in the hope of scoring a goal: a trim new *you!* By *no* means should this race extend to a competition with your friends. It will only cause you unhappiness if you are not 'ahead', and it just does not matter if Sue Bloggs down the road can run farther or appears to be slimming more rapidly. We are all different and therefore we all slim, flatten and trim at different speeds. Tension and pressure that result from competition detract from the pleasure of exercise and eventually defeat your purpose. Aerobic activity should be positive, not worrisome!

7. Take care of your feet. Do some research and buy a decent pair of shoes. Please! I cannot emphasise this enough. Be sure you purchase a pair designed

	DAYS 1–7	DAYS 8–14	DAYS 15–21	DAYS 22–30
NOVICE	Concentrate on pushing yourself when doing *any* walking: to the office, to the shops, with the dogs in the park. Feel the pull in the quadriceps and hamstrings as you strut at high speed. Try running a few laps around the block. Get the feel of what a good run can do for you. You want to *like* running, so break yourself in slowly. Supplement this with a try at the Aerobic Dance Routine outlined on page 58.	This week, take three runs. Pick any days you like! Probably weekend is the best time. The first two runs should be a full ¼ mile. The third must be ½ a mile. Time yourself. Also, do not slack off on the Aerobic Dance Routine. You should be giving it at least 1 hour a week. Add 2–5 minutes, perhaps one more song in your musical sequence.	You are now ready for your first mile. Map out an area that is exactly one mile, and try to complete the entire circuit. If you have to stop, keep walking briskly. Breathe deeply until the heartbeat returns to a normal pace, but do not stop moving. Once you feel up to it, start jogging again and complete the mile. Try this twice a week. You should then go on a third run of a length of your choice. Be smart: do *not* overdo it, but do not cheat yourself either. Complete the Aerobic Dance Routine 3 times this week.	This is the week to crystallise your aerobic routine. Do not think that just because this guide ends here, this should be the end of your training. Keeping fit is a continuous process. Now that you are beginning to see the changes and benefits, do not give up. Try 4 runs this week, at least 3 of these should be a mile. Do not forget your fast walking (this should be habit by now) and dancing. Make sure you perform some sort of aerobic exercise *every day!*
KEEN	You are going to begin with a concentrated effort to complete some sort of aerobic routine *every single day*. This can either be fast walking, jogging, the Aerobic Dance Routine as outlined on page 58, or some other sport of your choice. Run a full mile at least once this week.	Having broken yourself in a bit, you are ready to begin working. Jog 3 times this week. At least one of these runs should be over 1½ miles. Use your imagination and map out a route of this length. Add another 5 minutes to your Aerobic Dance Routine. And at least twice this week complete both a dancing and a running or walking routine. Feel those lungs expanding.	This week, go for a run or race-walk *every day*. Push yourself, you can take it now. Do not be afraid of a bit of discomfort. Try a 2-mile circuit.	With a friend, try a mini-marathon this week. Map out a route of at least 4 miles. This is probably further than you ever ran before, but do not panic. You are going to concentrate on *completing* the circuit. If you need to stop and walk for a while, *do* so, but keep moving and resume running as soon as you can. You can probably go further than you had imagined, but do not be stupid and overdo it. Also, double the length of time you spend on your other aerobic routines. And on day 30, why not try that 4-mile route again. Maybe you can run the whole way this time.

The 30-day aerobic routine based around jogging.

for training, not competition. Be wary of 'gimmick' shoes such as those with air-filled soles. Good designs have adequate arch support, elevated heels to relieve tendon strain, cushioned soles with nibs and a snug fit with plenty of toe-room.

8.   Relax and enjoy yourself!

For those of you who need a little encouragement to get started with aerobics, I have made up a chart (see page 57) which sets out a typical thirty-day aerobic routine for the novice and keen person based around jogging. Jogging, however, can be substituted for any other form of aerobic exercise, such as swimming, cycling or dancing.

I have not included a routine for the expert fitness trainer, since no dout you will already be an aerobic freak!

The aerobic dance routine

This routine can be done anywhere at any time. Be sure to pick a place where you feel comfortable and have plenty of room. You do not want to feel constrained at all. For this reason, wear loose, comfortable clothing. A leotard and tights or shorts and loose tee-shirt are the best for easy movement. Running shoes are beneficial, but not necessary. If you choose to complete the routine bare-footed, make sure you do not run on your toes the entire time. Roll the foot like you do when walking or running. This gives the heel and tendons a good stretch, lessening the chance of contracting shin splints or other foot/leg debilities.

Now all you need is some lively music and you are ready to begin. Turn on the tunes, shake out the legs, let loose and 'GO!'

1.   Assume starting position with straight back, pelvis

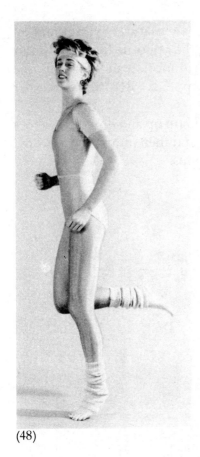 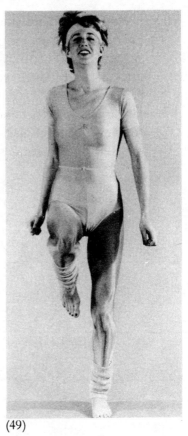

(48)   (49)

forward and stomach held in tight. Take two deep breaths, exhaling and inhaling deeply.

2. Lift feet off the ground one at a time and begin softly jogging on the spot.
3. Increase speed and vigour as the jog continues.
4. Kick up feet behind you and connect with buttock. Return to regular jogging (48).
5. Now lift legs high in front of you, knees bent, Russian-style (49). Keep this up as long as you can, then return to regular jogging. Be sure you are breathing properly.

59

6. Swing legs side to side, alternating, by jumping on one foot and throwing the opposite foot into the air sideways. Add some arm motion and turn this one into a wild dance step (50). Return to regular jogging action.

7. Bring feet together and hop up and down from toes to heels. Jump in place and then jump forward for 2 steps and back for 2 steps.

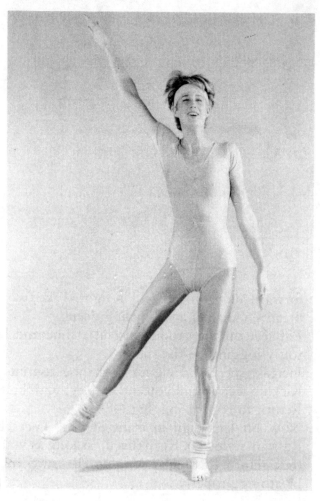

(50)

8. Keeping legs and knees together, jump side to side, alternating on each count. Then jump left for 2 counts and right for 2 counts.
9. Twist legs and lower body side to side. Make sure legs are tightly squeezed together (51). As you continue hopping, bend knees and lower body to floor. This is a great exercise for ski conditioning. Straighten up slowly. Keep hopping.
10. Now open legs and twist. Add arm swings.

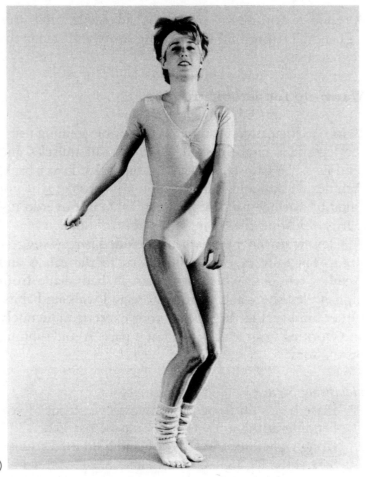

(51)

Lower body to floor and then straighten, maintaining control. Return to regular jogging.
11. Bring arms above head and inhale deeply, concentrating on filling the lungs. Exhale. Repeat.
12. Slow down your jogging on the spot. Continue breathing deeply.
13. Gradually decelerate your run until you are just bending the legs one after the other. Allow your heart rate to return to normal.

A good warm-down stretch is advisable after this sequence. Try one of the hamstring stretches listed in the next section.

Warm-up for aerobic training

Before participating in any kind of aerobic training using the legs, it is vital to stretch out the calf muscles and tendons. The hamstrings, calves, buttocks, lower back, Achilles tendon and feet can give you problems if not suitably warmed up. But be careful. Do not overdo it – learn to push to the 'point of no return' only.

A few warm-up exercises are included here as suggestions. They are especially beneficial to the calves and Achilles tendons, which are often in bad shape from high-heeled shoes and poor posture and walking habits. Other hints include beginning your exercise moderately and working up gradually to a faster pace. Avoid running on the toes.

Hamstring Stretch
1. Place hands on floor about two feet in front of you bending at the hip. Heels should be flat (52).
2. Bring right knee towards you and hold for 5 counts. Straighten leg (53).

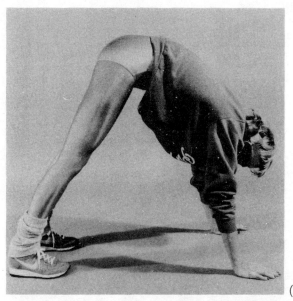

(52)

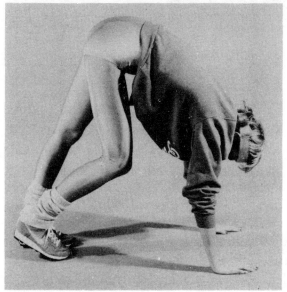

(53)

3. Bring left knee in and hold for 5 counts.
4. *Repeat*, alternating legs.

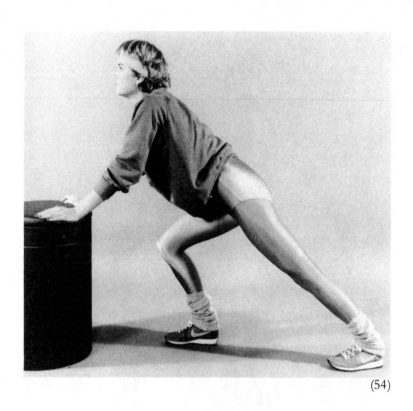

(54)

Calf and Tendon Stretch
1. Place hands on anything upright: tree, fence, wall. Bend right leg and place left leg back in a lunge keeping knee straight.
2. Strive to place heel on ground while keeping leg straight. Press firmly but carefully onto heel, stretching the Achilles tendon and back of calf (54). Hold for 10 counts.
3. Change legs and *repeat*. Be careful not to bounce into heel.

This is not a diet book and for that reason discussion of food intake will be kept to a minimum. It cannot, however, be left out altogether as no slimming or training programme is complete without a complementary routine of sensible eating.

Advice on diet is the final part of my three-part plan. To trim successfully your waist and thighs and flatten your stomach, you must combine exercising with a sensible diet – one just does not work without the other.

Like exercise, a controlled diet teaches the pleasures of discipline. You feel better, both physically and mentally if you are eating the right foods and in the right amounts. You will no longer turn down lunch dates or country weekends for fear of not being able to fit into your clothes the following day.

Diet and exercise are physiologically integrated. You live in a body that is fuelled by food, so you must eat to move. What actually happens is that when carbohydrates are ingested, they trigger a process of combustion within the body cells. The carbohydrates and oxygen 'burn' together to create energy, and this energy is measured in calories. The amount of exercise we do is directly proportional to the amount of calories we burn. Thus, to lose weight, you *must* decrease food intake, thereby decreasing the amount of calories taken in, while simultaneously increasing physical activity, thereby increasing the amount of calories used up. In this way, you begin to use stored fat cells as energy instead of lunch-time's chocolate cake, and the weight begins to drop off.

You *must* understand the basic principle behind a diet

before undertaking to follow one through. Once you have learned the principle and applied it, you will begin to see slimming results. It is only a marathon swimmer or a sugar-cane cutter who loses much weight through exercise alone. And it is foolish to diet without exercising – you can lose as much muscle as fat and find yourself permanently weakened if you neglect to tone and strengthen as well as reduce.

Contrary to what most people think, vigorous exercise actually depresses the appetite. Only light, moderate exercise may stimulate the desire to eat. The physical reason behind this is that exercise raises the blood sugar level, a metabolic signal of the need for satiation. Muscles use more fat than sugar so that this level becomes stabilised, a state that lasts a long time after you have finished exercising. So, you continue burning extra calories hours after your jog or squash game. Also, blood usually feeding into the gustatory system has been diverted into tendons and muscles. This lowers the desire for food. Exercise makes food pass through the gustatory system faster, so that instead of being stored, calories are burned as they pass.

Psychologically, exercise contributes to the maintenance of a diet. Having spent an hour or so working-out vigorously, you feel less inclined to undo all that 'good' and are able to resist that after-work pint which you used to feel was absolutely necessary to wind down. If you rethink your approach to body maintenance and combine an exercise routine with sensible eating, you will find you need never follow a formal diet again.

On the other hand, there is nothing wrong with a strict, regimented diet, as long as it is a healthy one, but most of the fashionable diets that appear in books and magazines are unhealthy. Just because they develop a popular following does not mean that they are safe or effective. Be especially wary of those diets that claim if you stick with them for two weeks, you can eat the way you want for the rest of your life.

Some of these diets fill you so full of protein that you will be unable to defecate properly, as well as dangerously depriving you of carbohydrates. At the same time, a vegetarian diet can deprive you of proteins, the body's building blocks. The only healthy vegetarian diet is one that includes plenty of nuts, soya and other proteins. The best type of diet is one that includes unrefined carbohydrates in moderation (whole grains), animal protein and a small amount of fat. In order to lose weight safely, you need to cut down your intake of *all* these foods, so that a balance – in miniature – is maintained.

Diet plans can work, but they take time – a month is the very least amount of time in which you can expect results.

Before you start a diet regime, understand your reasons for doing so. Just because your best friend is eating nothing but bean sprouts and bananas does not mean that you have to do the same. Be wary of the competition trap. So your sister is thinner than you – but she's not *you*. Only try to lose weight if *you* really have the need or genuine desire. Perhaps all you really need to do is straighten out a few bad habits.

First, assess your eating habits. Do you deny, then indulge? Do you nibble your way up the scales? Are you a closet eater? Take an honest look at your waistline and at your refrigerator-door habits (how many times a day do *you* open it?). Measure the amount of salad dressing you put on your 'low-calorie' salad. Think about how you fool yourself into believing you are cutting down ('just *one* chocolate'). View clearly what you are *really* doing. Then change the destructive habits to constructive ones.

A controlled diet takes considerable concentration and

effort and extraordinary discipline. You must realise that only hard work gains results. You must be prepared every single day for temptations. Get to know yourself. Learn what destructive pressures you give in to, and then do not allow yourself to fall into similar situations. At the same time, do not feel overly depressed or guilty if you 'break' once in a while. You are only human after all. It is important that you stay positive.

Now find a reduced-calorie scheme that suits your personality. This is best dictated by a doctor. Books and magazines can provide you with a legitimate plan, too, but remember what I said about fad diets. Adopt a pro-gramme to suit *you*. If you are the type that has a hard time sticking to diets, you had better stay away from activities focused on food for a while. Skip the dinner parties until you gain the strength to say 'no'.

Be realistic about your weight loss. Do not expect miracles. The slower the process of slimming, the more permanent it will be. An attitude develops in time, so be patient.

Beware of many of the fallacies spread by so-called diet experts and the media. Some of the Get-Thin-Quick ideas and devices are dangerous as well as non-produc-tive (and expensive). These include cellulite massage, laxatives/diuretics, starch 'blockers', saunas and steam-rooms, 'sweating off' inches via rubberised clothing, amphetamine diet pills, shake machines and hypnosis. Some of these reduce tension and help the muscles relax (often only the sphincters) which will aid you in sticking to a diet, but they are completely ineffective for body control or maintenance. Only a sensible diet combined with exercise will work.

Never starve yourself to lose weight quickly. A fright-ening condition which has become all too common, is anorexia nervosa. The person afflicted becomes disgusted by food and can literally starve to death. Another syndrome is bulemia: here the victim voluntarily vomits after eating, which can lead to the degeneration of vital body systems including the gustatory, enzymatic and excretory systems.

And it is especially important to keep yourself strong while you are undertaking an exercise programme.

Weakness caused by lower calorie intake can be compensated by making those calories you *do* consume, quality calories. A 250-calorie chocolate ice-cream gives you a temporary energy boost, a 'high' that lasts maybe half an hour, but it then leaves you empty. Complex foods such as fruit and vegetables (a banana, two apples and a 3-ounce slice of cheese is 250 calories) stay with you longer, giving you energy all day. Do not drastically reduce salt intake either. True, salt causes water retention, but the body needs that water, especially when you are active. Dehydration causes fatigue and headaches. Be sure you are eating for nourishment and sustenance.

A comprehensive slimming programme should not leave you apathetic or fiesty, but fit and vital.

I have included a list of eating tips, which I hope will get you started in the right direction.

1. *Never* skip meals. Shape an eating programme that fits your lifestyle. This may be from only two to as many as six small meals a day. Eat at the prescribed times only. If you are not hungry, try to eat something – no matter how small – so that you will not be absolutely famished at the next meal. Never eat in between meals.

2. Drink plenty of liquids. Low-calorie drinks such as decaffinated coffee, tea, diet sodas, mineral water and unsweetened fruit juice fill you up without filling you out.

3. Beware of hidden sugars in prepared foods. Learn to read labels. Foods like tomato sauce, tomato soup and fruit sauce are nearly all sugar, a fact easily obtained by scanning the fine print.

4. Do not buy fattening food or leave such foods lying around your house. Throw away the leftover pudding from your dinner party and spare your waistline.

5. Always sit down to eat a proper meal. That way you notice what you consume. Never eat a meal while standing in front of the refrigerator.

6. Do not 'pick' or nibble. There is something psychological about not putting a slice of cake on your plate, but you will probably eat twice as much if you pick at your boyfriend's.

7. Beware of alcohol. It contains calories with absolutely no nutritional value. Also, alcohol tends to relax you and can encourage you to eat foods you would not otherwise want.

8. Substitute low-fat foods for high-fat foods. Eat raw vegetables or fruit as a snack instead of crisps or nuts. Eat popcorn if you simply *must* have a salty snack. A cup of unpopped popcorn, prepared without butter, is only 50 calories.

9. Do not lavish butter or creamy spreads on your otherwise 'low-calorie' meat, salads or vegetables.

10. Always leave something behind on your plate.

11. Be sure to eat breakfast every day, even if it is only a very light meal. This prevents you from hungrily consuming the entire bread basket at lunch-time as you wait for your meal to arrive. I suggest you try my 'California Breakfast', which is high in nutrients, bulk and proteins but low in calories. The recipe is below.

12. Eat slowly and carefully. Be the last to finish, so that

you are not tempted to try a 'bite' of other people's dinners.

As promised, here is the recipe for my 'California Breakfast'. After your morning exercise and before work, this meal is a fantastic energiser. It has its origins in a wetsuit-strewn apartment in Isla Vista, California, overlooking the Pacific surf. It is quick and easy to prepare, and can be a lot of fun too as you can use your imagination when mixing together the ingredients. It only contains nutritive calories so, although the meal can be large, it will not add weight.

You will need:

1 carton low-fat natural yoghurt
1 cup pure grain cereal or non-sweetened granola (I recommend Grapenuts)
fresh fruit of your choice (apples, bananas, nectarines, strawberries are the best, but any will do)
sultanas, currents or raisins
wheatgerm or bran

Combine all the ingredients in a bowl with a little milk. Dig in and enjoy! You could vary the dish by using other ingredients found in your cupboard. Sunflower seeds or coconut slices add lots of flavour – but be careful of adding too many calories!

More Dieting Tips
An extra dieting tip is to keep your diet a secret. By not telling anyone you eliminate the need to justify your actions and the guilt that often accompanies them. It relieves you from having to deal with a sort of psychological sabotage from other people, one that is motivated by jealousy, insecurity or simply naiveté. Also, the concept of 'diet' often denotes failure in other people's eyes,

so deny that this is what you are doing. Your 'food control' must become a special part of your life, one that will help you with your self-image. You will gain great personal satisfaction when someone compliments you on how wonderful you look. And you will smile mysteriously and tell them that this colour always suited you. Besides, it is *incredibly* boring to discuss dieting constantly .

Another tip is just the opposite. Let *everyone* know you are dieting. In this way you trap yourself into either succeeding or being humiliated. This only works for certain types of people, those who can stand – even thrive on – such pressure.

Some people find that allowing themselves one goodie a week helps them 'stay good' the rest of the week. This means that once a week you sit down with a bowl of chocolate ice-cream or a piece of apple pie. You watch yourself consume the entire fattening substance, fully conscious of your actions. This will not only leave you sweet-satiated, but also slightly guilty (guilt in small doses can work positively) so that you will be less likely to indulge in the days to come.

Probably the best tip of all is to take your diet *one day at a time*. As with your exercise routine, do not worry about tomorrow. Complete what you have to do today to the best of your ability and then forget about it. Get on with your life! A body maintenance programme is aimed at keeping your machinery running healthily and smoothly so that you do not have to worry or even think about it. Quality existence is what you are striving for!

NOVICE (*number of repetitions to be performed for each exercise*)

Day	Leg lunges	Waist pulls & twists	Leg lifts	More leg lifts	Fire hydrant lifts	Bun burners	Open leg stretches	Stomach strengtheners	Sit-ups	Leg extensions	Raised leg sequence	Scissors
1	4	4	4	4	2	4	4	4	8	8	8	4
2	4	4	4	4	2	4	4	4	8	8	8	4
3	4	4	4	4	2	4	4	4	8	12	8	4
4	4	4	4	4	2	4	4	4	12	12	8	4
5	4	4	4	4	2	4	4	4	12	12	12	4
6	4	4	4	4	2	4	4	4	12	12	12	8
7	4	4	4	8	2	4	4	4	12	16	12	8
8	4	4	8	8	3	8	8	4	12	16	12	8
9	4	8	8	8	3	8	8	8	16	16	12	8
10	8	8	8	8	3	8	8	8	16	16	12	8
11	8	8	8	8	3	8	8	8	16	16	16	8
12	8	8	8	8	4	8	8	8	16	16	16	8
13	8	8	12	8	4	8	8	8	16	16	16	12
14	8	8	12	8	4	8	8	8	16	16	16	12
15	8	16	12	8	4	12	12	8	16	16	16	12

NOVICE (continued)

Day	Leg lunges	Waist pulls & twists	Leg lifts	More leg lifts	Fire hydrant lifts	Bun burners	Open leg stretches	Stomach strengtheners	Sit-ups	Leg extensions	Raised leg sequence	Scissors
16	8	16	12	8	4	12	12	8	16	20	16	12
17	12	16	12	8	5	12	12	12	20	20	16	12
18	12	16	12	12	5	12	12	12	20	20	20	12
19	12	20	12	12	5	12	12	12	20	20	20	12
20	12	20	12	12	6	12	12	12	20	20	20	12
21	12	20	12	12	6	12	12	12	20	20	20	12
22	12	20	12	12	6	12	12	12	20	20	20	16
23	12	24	12	12	7	12	12	16	20	24	24	16
24	16	24	12	12	7	12	16	16	20	24	24	16
25	16	24	16	12	7	12	16	16	24	24	24	16
26	16	30	16	16	7	16	16	16	24	24	24	16
27	16	30	16	16	8	16	16	16	24	24	24	16
28	16	30	16	16	8	16	16	16	24	24	30	16
29	16	40	16	16	8	16	16	16	24	24	30	16
30	20	40	20	20	12	20	20	20	30	30	30	16

KEEN (*number of repetitions to be performed for each exercise*)

Day	Leg lunges	Waist pulls & twists	Leg lifts	More leg lifts	Fire hydrant lifts	Bun burners	Open leg stretches	Stomach strengtheners	Sit-ups	Leg extensions	Raised leg sequence	Scissors
1	8	8	8	4	4	4	8	8	16	12	12	8
2	8	8	8	4	4	4	8	8	16	12	12	8
3	8	8	8	4	4	4	8	8	16	12	12	8
4	12	8	8	4	4	4	8	8	16	12	16	8
5	12	8	8	4	6	6	8	12	20	16	16	8
6	12	8	8	4	6	6	8	12	20	16	16	8
7	12	8	8	8	6	6	12	12	20	16	16	8
8	12	8	8	8	6	6	12	12	24	16	16	12
9	12	8	8	8	6	6	12	12	24	16	16	12
10	12	8	12	8	8	8	12	12	24	20	20	12
11	12	8	12	8	8	8	12	12	24	20	20	12
12	16	8	12	8	8	8	12	12	24	20	20	12
13	16	12	12	8	8	8	12	16	24	20	20	12
14	16	12	12	8	8	8	12	16	30	20	20	12
15	16	12	12	8	8	8	16	16	30	20	20	12

KEEN (continued)

Day	Leg lunges	Waist pulls & twists	Leg lifts	More leg lifts	Fire hydrant lifts	Bun burners	Open leg stretches	Stomach strengtheners	Sit-ups	Leg extensions	Raised leg sequence	Scissors
16	16	12	12	8	8	8	16	16	30	24	20	12
17	16	12	12	8	8	8	16	16	30	24	24	16
18	20	12	12	8	8	8	16	16	30	24	24	16
19	20	12	16	8	8	12	16	16	30	24	24	16
20	20	12	16	8	8	12	16	16	30	24	24	16
21	20	12	16	12	8	12	20	16	30	24	24	16
22	20	16	16	12	12	12	20	16	36	24	24	16
23	24	16	16	12	12	16	20	20	36	24	30	20
24	24	16	20	16	12	16	20	20	36	30	30	20
25	24	16	20	16	12	16	24	20	36	30	30	20
26	24	20	20	16	12	20	24	20	36	30	30	24
27	24	20	24	20	12	20	24	20	36	30	30	24
28	24	20	24	20	12	20	24	24	40	30	36	24
29	24	24	24	20	12	24	24	24	40	36	36	24
30	30	24	30	24	16	24	30	30	40	36	36	24

EXPERT (*number of repetitions to be performed for each exercise*)

Day	Leg lunges	Waist pulls & twists	Leg lifts	More leg lifts	Fire hydrant lifts	Bun burners	Open leg stretches	Stomach strengtheners	Sit-ups	Leg extensions	Raised leg sequence	Scissors
1	8	12	12	8	8	8	12	12	16 situps only	2 × 12	16	16
2	8	12	12	8	8	8	12	12	16	2	16	16
3	12	12	12	8	8	8	12	12	20	2	16	16
4	12	16	12	8	8	12	12	16	20	2	16	16
5	12	16	16	8	12	12	12	16	20	3	20	16
6	12	16	16	12	12	12	12	16	24	3	20	20
7	12	16	16	12	12	12	16	20	24	3	20	20
8	16	16	16	12	12	12	16	20	24	3	20	20
9	16	16	20	12	12	12	16	20	30	3	20	20
10	16	16	20	12	12	12	16	20	30	4	20	20
11	16	16	20	12	16	12	16	24	30	4	20	20
12	16	16	20	12	16	12	16	24	30	4	24	24
13	16	16	24	16	16	16	20	24	40	4	24	24
14	16	20	24	16	16	16	20	24	40	4	24	24
15	20	20	24	16	16	16	20	24	44	4	24	24

EXPERT (*continued*)

Day	Leg lunges	Waist pulls & twists	Leg lifts	More leg lifts	Fire hydrant lifts	Bun burners	Open leg stretches	Stomach strengtheners	Sit-ups	Leg extensions	Raised leg sequence	Scissors
16	20	20	24	16	20	16	20	24	50	4	30	30
17	20	24	24	20	20	16	24	30	50	4	30	30
18	20	24	30	20	20	16	24	30	50	5	30	30
19	24	24	30	20	24	16	24	30	50	5	30	30
20	24	24	30	24	24	20	24	30	50	5	30	30
21	24	24	30	24	24	20	30	30	50	5	30	30
22	24	24	30	24	24	20	30	30	55	5	36	36
23	24	24	30	24	24	20	30	36	55	5	36	36
24	24	30	36	24	24	24	30	36	55	6	36	36
25	24	30	36	30	30	24	36	36	55	6	36	36
26	30	30	36	30	30	24	36	36	60	6	36	40
27	30	36	36	30	30	24	36	36	60	8	40	40
28	30	36	40	30	30	24	40	40	60	8	40	40
29	30	36	40	30	36	30	40	40	60	12	40	40
30	30	40	40	30	36	30	40	40	60	12	40	40